ABC OF SEXUALLY TRANSMITTED INFECTIONS

Fifth Edition

ABC OF SEXUALLY TRANSMITTED INFECTIONS

Fifth Edition

Michael Adler, Frances Cowan, Patrick French,
Helen Mitchell, and John Richens
Department of Sexually Transmitted Diseases,
Royal Free and University College Medical School
London

© BMJ Publishing Group Ltd 1984, 1990, 1995, 1998, 2004

First published in 1984 as *ABC of Sexually Transmitted Diseases*.
This fifth edition published in 2004 as ABC of Sexually Transmitted Infections by
BMJ Publishing Group Ltd, BMA House Tavistock Square, London WC1H 9JR

First Edition 1984
Second Edition 1990
Third Edition 1995
Fourth Edition 1998
Second Impression 2000
Third Impression 2001
Fifth Edition 2004
www.bmjbooks.com

British Library Cataloguing in Publication Data

A catalogue record for this book is available from the British Library

ISBN 0 7279 17617

Typeset by Newgen Imaging Systems (P) Ltd., Chennai, India
Printed and bound by GraphyCems, Navarra

The cover design is a false colour transmission electron
micrograph (TEM) of a cluster of the bacteria, *Chlamydia trachomatis*
with permission from Alfred Pasieka/Science Photo Library

Contents

Contributors   vi

Preface   vii

1 **Why sexually transmitted infections are important**   1
Michael Adler

2 **Control and prevention**   7
Frances Cowan

3 **The clinical process**   11
Patrick French

4 **Examination techniques and clinical sampling**   15
Patrick French

5 **Main presentations of sexually transmitted infections in male patients**   17
John Richens

6 **Other conditions of the male genital tract commonly seen in sexually transmitted infection clinics**   21
John Richens

7 **Vaginal discharge—causes, diagnosis, and treatment**   25
Helen Mitchell

8 **Pelvic inflammatory disease and pelvic pain**   30
Helen Mitchell

9 **Sexually transmitted infections in pregnancy**   34
Helen Mitchell

10 **Other conditions that affect the female genital tract**   39
Helen Mitchell

11 **Genital ulcer disease**   44
Frances Cowan

12 **Syphilis—clinical features, diagnosis, and management**   49
Michael Adler, Patrick French

13 **Genital growths**   56
Michael Adler

14 **Genital infestations**   60
Michael Adler

15 **Viral hepatitis**   62
Richard Gilson

16 **HIV**   68
Ian G Williams, Ian Weller

17 **Laboratory diagnosis of sexually transmitted infections**   80
Beryl West

Appendix. proformas for taking sexual histories   85

Index   87

Contributors

Michael Adler
Professor, Department of Sexually Transmitted Diseases, Royal Free and University College Medical School, London

Frances Cowan
Senior Lecturer, Department of Sexually Transmitted Diseases, Royal Free and University College Medical School, London

Patrick French
Consultant Physician in Genitourinary Medicine, Honorary Senior Lecturer, Department of Sexually Transmitted Diseases, Royal Free and University College Medical School, London

Richard Gilson
Senior Lecturer, Department of Sexually Transmitted Diseases, Royal Free and University College Medical School, London

Helen Mitchell
Consultant Physician in Sexual and Reproductive Health, Honorary Senior Lecturer, Department of Sexually Transmitted Diseases, Royal Free and University College Medical School, London

John Richens
Lecturer, Department of Sexually Transmitted Diseases, Royal Free and University College Medical School, London

Ian Weller
Professor, Department of Sexually Transmitted Diseases, Royal Free and University College Medical School, London

Beryl West
Medical Research Council Laboratories, Banjul, Gambia

Ian G Williams
Senior Lecturer, Department of Sexually Transmitted Diseases, Royal Free and University College Medical School, London

Preface

The first edition of this book appeared 20 years ago, virtually as a single author effort. This fifth edition comes at a time when the burden of sexually transmitted infections and HIV is at its greatest, yet and with an increasing importance of viral sexually acquired infections and new diagnostic tests. I am delighted that the fifth edition, and first of the new millennium, is now multi-author, written with colleagues from the Royal Free and University College. We have tried to capture recent advances at the same time as remaining practical with different approaches to control, diagnosis, and management depending on resources and facilities available.

Michael Adler,
London 2004

1 Why sexually transmitted infections are important

Michael Adler

What are sexually transmitted infections?

Sexually transmitted infections (STIs) are infections whose primary route of transmission is through sexual contact. STIs can be caused by mainly bacteria, viruses, or protozoa. In the developed world, viral diseases have become increasingly common and important, whereas bacterial STIs are more common in developing countries, but even this is changing with the increasing recognition of viral diseases.

The three most common presenting symptoms of an STI are urethral discharge, genital ulceration, and vaginal discharge with or without vulval irritation. The three most common STIs seen in clinics in the United Kingdom are genital warts, chlamydial infections, and gonococcal infections. Trichomoniasis, pediculosis pubis, and genital herpes are common and are sexually transmitted. Scabies and vaginal candidiasis often are diagnosed in STI clinics, although they are not usually acquired sexually. Finally, sexually transmitted hepatitis (A, B, and C) and HIV are becoming more common.

Why STIs are important

- Common
- Often asymptomatic
- Major complications and sequelae
- Expensive
- Synergy with HIV

Sexually transmitted infections and associated presenting symptoms

	Urethral discharge	Vaginal discharge	Genital ulceration	Skin symptoms	Other
Bacteria					
Chlamydia trachomatis	++	+/−			
Neisseria gonorrhoeae	++	+/−			
Treponema pallidum			++	+	+
Gardnerella vaginalis	+/−	++			
Haemophilus ducreyi			++		
Klebsiella granulomatis			++		
Shigella					+
Mycoplasmas					
Ureaplasma urealyticum	+				
Mycoplasma genitalium	+	+			+
Parasites					
Sarcoptes scabiei				+	
Phthirus pubis				+	
Viruses					
Herpes simplex virus types 1 and 2	(+)	(+)	++		
Wart virus (papillomavirus)	(+)	(+)		+	+
Molluscum contagiosum (pox virus)				+	
Hepatitis A, B, and C					+
HIV				+	++
Protozoa					
Entamoeba histolytica					+
Giardia lamblia					+
Trichomonas vaginalis	(+)	++			
Fungi					
Candida albicans	(+)	++			

+ Common. − Less common

1

The consequences

Sexually transmitted infections are a major public health problem and are one of the most common causes of illness, and even death, in the world today. They have far reaching health, social, and economic consequences, particularly in the developing world. The World Bank estimated that for women aged 15-44 years, STIs (excluding HIV) were the second most common cause of healthy life lost after maternal morbidity. Other studies have estimated that 5% of the total discounted healthy life years lost in sub-Saharan Africa are caused by STIs, excluding HIV, and that HIV alone accounts for 10% of healthy life years lost.

Complications and cost

Most STIs are easy to diagnose and cheap to treat; however, viral conditions, such as herpes and HIV, are costly and incurable. Many infections remain unrecognised and undiagnosed, which results in considerable long term morbidity, which can be costly in human and monetary terms. The complications of untreated infections are far reaching, and include cancer, reproductive problems, and pregnancy related problems. Reproductive ill health (death and disability related to pregnancy and childbirth, STIs, HIV, AIDS, and reproductive cancers) has been calculated to account for 5-15% of the global burden of disease. Data on the monetary costs of the complications of STIs are sparse, particularly for the developing world. American data give estimates of total direct and indirect costs attributable to STIs to be $9.9 m annually, rising to $16.6 m if HIV and AIDS are included. In the United Kingdom only limited data are available. For example, the prevention of unplanned pregnancy by NHS contraception services probably saves over £2.5 billion per year, and the average lifetime treatment cost for an HIV positive person is between £135 000 and £180 000, with a monetary value of preventing a single onward transmission of somewhere between £0.5 m to £1 m in terms of individual health benefits and treatment costs. Finally, but not calculated accurately, dramatic cost savings can be made by preventing infertility.

Few economic data exist in the developing world in relation to the consequences of STIs, which are considerable and personally devastating. Many women become infertile without even realising that they have suffered from pelvic inflammatory disease. Estimates of the burden of infections for women in urban Africa have shown that chlamydial infection causes an average of 4.8 lost days of productive life and syphilis leads to 8.2 days per capita per year. Estimates suggest that with the high prevalence of syphilis in pregnant women, for example 10%, up to 8% of all pregnancies (beyond 12 weeks) would have an adverse outcome.

Synergy between STIs and HIV

It is now recognised that there is a synergy between most STIs and HIV (particularly ulcerative and inflammatory conditions). Many research studies in both the developed and developing world have shown that HIV transmission and acquisition are enhanced by the presence of STIs, probably because of the inflammatory effect of STIs in the genital mucosa. HIV negative people with an ulcerative STI seem to be particularly vulnerable to infection, probably because in addition to the genital inflammation that occurs, ulceration causes physical disruption of the skin or mucous membrane, thus making it more permeable to infection. Non-ulcerative STIs also facilitate HIV acquisition and transmission but to a lesser degree. As they are

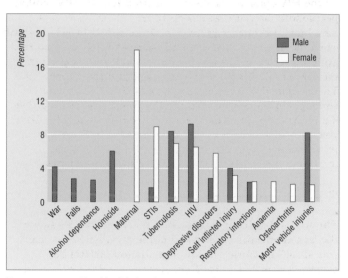

Top ten causes of healthy life lost in young adults aged 15-44 years

Major sequelae of STIs

	Women	Men	Infants
Cancers	Cervical cancer Vulval cancer Vaginal cancer Anal cancer Liver cancer T cell leukaemia Kaposi's sarcoma	Penile cancer Anal cancer Liver cancer T cell leukaemia Kaposi's sarcoma	
Reproductive health problems	Pelvic inflammatory disease Infertility Ectopic pregnancy Spontaneous abortion	Epididymitis Prostatitis Infertility	
Pregnancy related problems	Preterm delivery Premature rupture of membranes Puerperal sepsis Postpartum infection		Stillbirth Low birth weight Pneumonia Neonatal sepsis Acute hepatitis Congenital abnormalities
Neurological problems	Neurosyphilis	Neurosyphilis	Cytomegalo-virus Herpes simplex virus Syphilis associated neurological problems
Other common health consequences	Chronic liver disease Cirrhosis	Chronic liver disease Cirrhosis	Chronic liver disease Cirrhosis

so common in many parts of the world, however, their impact on the HIV epidemic is likely to be considerable. HIV positive people with intercurrent ulcerative and non-ulcerative STIs have increased rates of genital shedding of HIV, which diminish when the STI is resolved. Clinical studies have shown that HIV positive patients with a urethral infection have an eightfold increase in HIV-1 RNA in semen, which falls after treatment. The likelihood of infection per exposure to HIV for any sexual contact is in the order of 0.1, which will increase considerably if an STI is present by the order of threefold to fivefold. This synergy, and a realisation that the control of STIs can have a profound effect on the incidence of HIV, has led to an increased drive and interest in STI control programmes.

Size of the problem

The size of the global burden of STIs is uncertain because of the lack of effective control and notification systems in many countries. The World Health Organization (WHO) has estimated a total of 340 million new cases of curable STIs in adults per annum, mainly in South and South East Asia (151 million new cases per year), and sub-Saharan Africa (69 million). In eastern Europe and Central Asia, the estimate is 22 million, and 17 million in western Europe. The prevalence and incidence per million of the population varies regionally, for example between sub-Saharan Africa and western Europe it is eightfold and fourfold, respectively.

Role of STIs in the acquisition of HIV

- HIV acquisition increases by twofold to fivefold in the presence of other STIs
- Ulcers disrupt mucosal integrity and increase the presence or activation, or both, of HIV susceptible cells (for example, CD4 lymphocytes)
- Non-ulcerative STIs (such as gonorrhoea, chlamydia, *Trichomonas vaginalis*, and bacterial vaginosis) increase the presence or activation, or both, of HIV susceptible cells

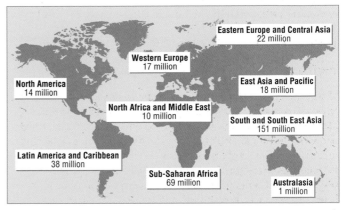

Estimated new cases of curable STIs among adults (global total 340 million). Data source: World Health Organization

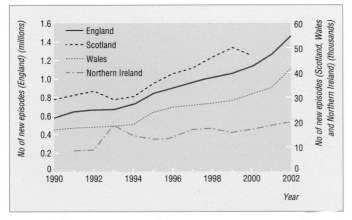

All diagnoses and workload at genitourinary medicine clinics by country, 1990-2002. Data are unavailable currently for Scotland for 2000-2 and Northern Ireland for 1990. Adapted from slide from Health Protection Agency (www.hpa.org.uk), Communicable Disease Surveillance Centre. Data from KC60 statutory returns and ISD(D)5 data

New diagnoses of selected STIs in GUM clinics (England, Wales, and Northern Ireland, 2002)

	2002	% change 1996-2002
Chlamydia	81 680	139
Genital warts	69 417	17
Gonorrhoea	24 953	106
Genital herpes	18 392	16
Syphilis	1193	870

The United Kingdom has a network of clinics dealing with STIs (departments of genitourinary medicine (GUM)), and such clinics have seen a very substantial increase in the number of attendances over the past decade. Such attendances have doubled, reaching 1.5 million in the year 2002. Even in the last seven years, increases of over 100% have been seen in cases of chlamydia, gonorrhoea, and syphilis.

Gonorrhoea

To interpret differences between countries and even trends is difficult because of the variation in reporting practices and the provision of facilities. Rates of gonorrhoea vary between European countries. During the early to mid 1970s the number of cases of gonorrhoea peaked in most European countries. The subsequent advent of HIV and AIDS in the 1980s led to safer sexual practices and a reduction in the incidence of gonorrhoea, which has not been sustained in all countries. For example, between 1996 and 2002 an increase has been seen in both male and female cases of gonorrhoea in England

Estimated prevalence and incidence of STIs by region

Region	Prevalence per million	Incidence per million
Sub-Saharan Africa	32	69
South and South East Asia	48	151
Latin America and Caribbean	18.5	38
Eastern Europe and Central Asia	6	22
North America	3	14
Australasia	0.3	1
Western Europe	4	17
Northern Africa and Middle East	3.5	10
East Asia and Pacific	6	18
TOTAL	**116.5**	**340**

and Wales (114% increase in the number of cases in heterosexual men from 8051 to 17 260, and an 86% increase in cases in women from 4045 to 7542). The incidence of gonorrhoea has increased since 1996 in homosexual men, particularly in those living in London, as has that of other STIs. In 2002, 16% of gonorrhoea diagnoses in men, and 19% of those in London, were acquired through homosexual sex.

Other western European and Scandinavian countries have also seen recent increases, for example in France and Sweden. Eastern Europe, and particularly the newly independent states of the former Soviet Union, has seen an epidemic of STIs, with high rates of gonorrhoea in Estonia, Russia, and Belarus.

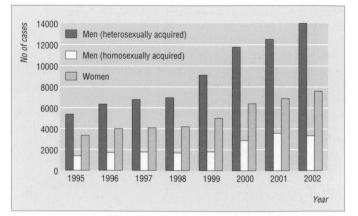

Cases of uncomplicated gonorrhoea seen in genitourinary medicine clinics by sex and male sexual orientation in England, Wales, and Northern Ireland, 1995-2002. Adapted from slide from Health Protection Agency (www.hpa.org.uk), Communicable Disease Surveillance Centre. Data from KC60 statutory returns

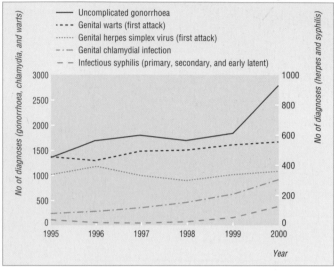

New diagnoses of selected STIs in men who have sex with men, England and Wales, 1995-2000. Adapted from slide from Health Protection Agency (www.hpa.org.uk), Communicable Disease Surveillance Centre

Syphilis

Syphilis is now rare in western Europe and North America, which is mainly due to the control of early acquired infectious syphilis in women and screening of pregnant women for syphilis. In most western European countries the incidence of syphilis has continued to decline to below five per 100 000. As mentioned above, an epidemic of most STIs has occurred in eastern Europe, with a recent epidemic of syphilis in all the newly independent states of the former Soviet Union. This epidemic is the vanguard of an HIV epidemic, and outbreaks of HIV have been reported in intravenous drug users, particularly in Belarus, Russia, and Ukraine. Likewise, syphilis is still a major clinical problem and a cause of genital ulceration in the developing world.

It is of concern that syphilis also is increasing again in the United Kingdom. In the past seven years, the cases of infectious syphilis have increased by 870%, particularly in men heterosexual and homosexual.

Chlamydia

Chlamydia is still a major public health problem in most of Europe and North America. In the United Kingdom, infection with *Chlamydia trachomatis* is now the most common curable bacterial STI. Since 1996 the number of cases has increased, with cases in women outnumbering cases in men. In 2002, 81 680 people with chlamydial infections attended clinics.

This condition is most commonly seen in young people; the peak age is between 20 and 24 years in men and between 16 and 19 years in women. Screening surveys performed outside normal STI clinic environments also show high levels in antenatal and gynaecology clinics, general practice, and family

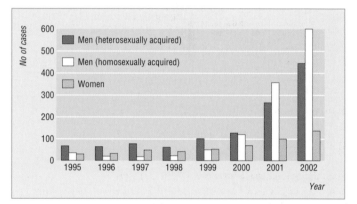

Cases of infectious syphilis (primary and secondary) seen in genitourinary medicine clinics by sex and male sexual orientation in England, Wales, and Northern Ireland, 1995-2002. Adapted from slide from Health Protection Agency (www.hpa.org.uk), Communicable Disease Surveillance Centre

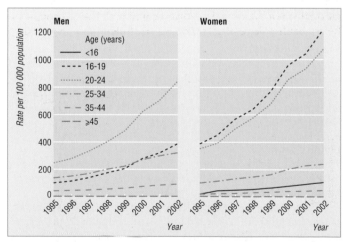

Diagnoses of uncomplicated genital chlamydial infection in genitourinary medicine clinics by sex and age group in the United Kingdom, 1995-2002. Data are unavailable for Scotland for 2000-2. Adapted from slide from Health Protection Agency (www.hpa.org.uk), Communicable Disease Surveillance Centre. Data from KC60 statutory returns and ISD(D)5 data

planning and pregnancy termination clinics, with the prevalence rate ranging from 4.5% to 12%.

Genital herpes and warts
Compared with gonorrhoea and chlamydia, the increase in cases of genital herpes and warts has slowed down in British GUM clinics in the past few years.

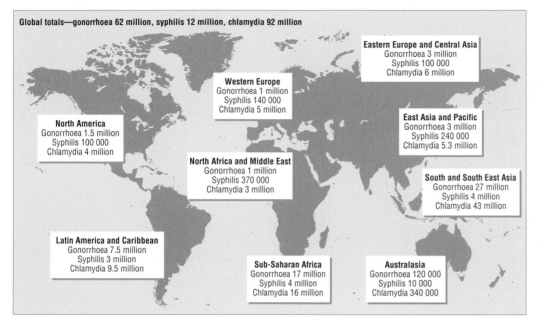

Global totals—gonorrhoea 62 million, syphilis 12 million, chlamydia 92 million

Eastern Europe and Central Asia
Gonorrhoea 3 million
Syphilis 100 000
Chlamydia 6 million

Western Europe
Gonorrhoea 1 million
Syphilis 140 000
Chlamydia 5 million

North America
Gonorrhoea 1.5 million
Syphilis 100 000
Chlamydia 4 million

East Asia and Pacific
Gonorrhoea 3 million
Syphilis 240 000
Chlamydia 5.3 million

North Africa and Middle East
Gonorrhoea 1 million
Syphilis 370 000
Chlamydia 3 million

South and South East Asia
Gonorrhoea 27 million
Syphilis 4 million
Chlamydia 43 million

Latin America and Caribbean
Gonorrhoea 7.5 million
Syphilis 3 million
Chlamydia 9.5 million

Sub-Saharan Africa
Gonorrhoea 17 million
Syphilis 4 million
Chlamydia 16 million

Australasia
Gonorrhoea 120 000
Syphilis 10 000
Chlamydia 340 000

Estimated new cases of the three most common STIs among adults

STIs in developing countries

Sexually transmitted infections have a much higher incidence and prevalence in developing countries and are among the top five reasons for consultation in general health services in many African countries. Routine and accurate surveillance data are often lacking, and an understanding of the burden of infection tends to come from WHO estimates and ad hoc surveys, usually in high risk groups.

Particularly high rates of infections are seen in groups such as female prostitutes and their clients and truck drivers. Prostitution continues to be an important factor in the transmission of STIs in developing countries. For example, in an urban Kenyan STI clinic, 60% of men with a diagnosis of gonorrhoea or chancroid reported commercial sex exposure as the probable source of infection. Genital ulcer disease is more

> **High rates of syphilis, chlamydia, and gonorrhoea are seen particularly in sub-Saharan Africa and South and South East Asia**

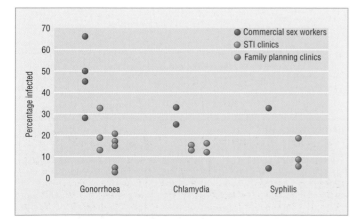

STIs in women in Africa

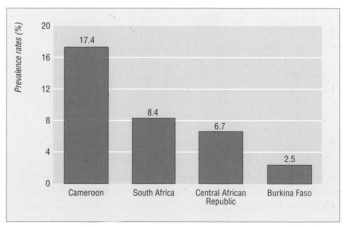

Syphilis prevalence rates (%) in pregnant women in Africa in 1990s

frequent in developing countries (syphilis, chancroid, lymphogranuloma venereum, and granuloma inguinale), and in sub-Saharan Africa, 20-70% of patients who attend clinics present with ulcers. In commercial sex workers, the prevalence of gonorrhoea can reach nearly 50%, and the prevalence of syphilis ranges from 2% to 30% for acute or previous infection. Infection with herpes simplex virus (type 2) is almost universal among commercial sex workers in various African countries, for example Zimbabwe. Rates of syphilis in women who attend antenatal clinics are high, with rates reaching 17% in Cameroon. Levels of chlamydia can be as high as 30%.

The incidence of STI complications and their sequelae is much higher in developing countries because of the lack of resources and adequate diagnosis and treatment. Particular complications are adverse pregnancy outcomes for mother and baby, neonatal and infant infections, infertility in both sexes, ectopic pregnancy, urethral strictures in males, and blindness in infants caused by gonococcal and chlamydial ophthalmia neonatorum and in adults caused by gonococcal keratoconjunctivitis, as well as genital cancers, particularly cancers of the cervix and penis.

Why are STIs increasing?

Like many other medicosocial conditions, for example suicide, alcoholism, cancer, and heart disease, the explanation for the increase is multi-factorial. Attitudes towards sex and sexual behaviour have changed. The survey of Sexual Attitudes and Lifestyle carried out in the United Kingdom plotted changes between 1990 and 2000.

- Age at first intercourse has declined, and half of all teenagers have sex before they are 17 years of age
- The number of lifetime male and female heterosexual partners has increased since 1990, with the highest increases in young people
- The proportion of men and women who have concurrent relationships (having more than one sexual partner at the same time) has increased
- Condom use has increased in the United Kingdom but may be offset by the increase in the number of sexual partners. For example, the proportion of the population who reported two or more partners in the past year and who did not use condoms consistently has increased since 1990 from 13.6% to 15.4% for men and from 7.1% to 10% for women
- The proportion of men in the United Kingdom who have ever had a homosexual partner in the last five years increased between 1990 and 2000. Unsafe sex in homosexual men has increased, particularly in London
- Populations are now more mobile nationally and internationally. Certain groups (tourists, professional travellers, members of the armed forces, and immigrants) are at risk. They are separated from their families and social restraints and are more likely to have sexual contact outside a stable relationship. In addition, poverty, urbanisation, war, and social migration often result in increased levels of prostitution.

Conclusion

Sexually transmitted infections are a major public health problem throughout the world, in terms of morbidity and mortality and in their facilitatory role in the acquisition and transmission of HIV. Prevention programmes are essential to deal with these issues (see Chapter 2).

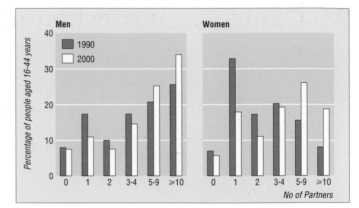

Percentage distribution of heterosexual partners in lifetime by sex, 1999 and 2000. Adapted from National Survey of Sexual Attitudes and Lifestyles, 2000

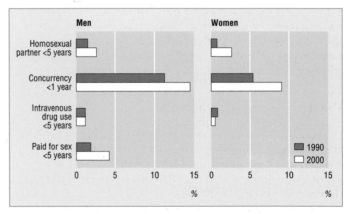

Changes in behaviour over time. Adapted from National Survey of Sexual Attitudes and Lifestyles, 2000

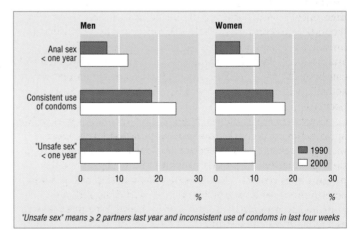

"Unsafe sex" means ≥ 2 partners last year and inconsistent use of condoms in last four weeks

Changes in behaviour over time. Adapted from National Survey of Sexual Attitudes and Lifestyles, 2000

Further reading

- Adler MW, Cowan FM. Sexually transmitted infections. In: Detek R, McEwen J, eds. *Oxford textbook of public health: the practice of public health.* 4th ed, vol 3. Oxford: Oxford University Press, 2002, pp 1441-52
- Adler M, Foster J, Grosskurth H, Richens J, Slavin H. *Sexual health and care: sexually transmitted infections, guidelines for prevention and treatment.* London: Overseas Development Administration, 1996

2   Control and prevention

Frances Cowan

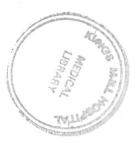

Sexually transmitted infections (STIs) represent one of the major public health problems in the world today, as outlined in Chapter 1. The demographic, sociological, economic, and behavioural changes seen throughout the world in the past 40 years will continue to drive the spread of STIs.

Pattern of spread

Several factors are known to be important in maintaining the spread of STIs in communities. A simple arithmetic formula has been developed that makes it possible to anticipate the pattern of spread of STIs in communities under certain circumstances. If the average number of infections that result from one infection is greater than one, then the rate of that STI will increase in the community. Conversely, if the average number of infections is less than one, then the rate of spread of the STI will fall. Reductions in any of these variables at a community level will decrease the average number of new infections that result from one infection in that community.

Principles of control

The approach to controlling STIs and the emphasis placed on different components will depend on the local pattern and distribution of STIs in the community and whether one is working in a setting that is resource rich or resource poor. However, the same general principles will apply.

Prevention can be aimed at uninfected people in the community to prevent them from acquiring infection (primary prevention) or at infected people to prevent the onward transmission of the infection to their sexual partners (secondary prevention). Although effective primary prevention can theoretically reduce the prevalence of viral and bacterial STIs, secondary prevention is much more effective at reducing the prevalence of bacterial STIs, which all are curable with antibiotics. In fact, the population prevalence of a bacterial STI can be reduced entirely through effective secondary prevention activities without any reduction in risky sexual behaviour occurring.

Countries that combine primary and secondary prevention approaches, at the individual and population levels, have managed substantially to reduce the burden of infection in their population. Effective implementation of prevention programmes requires strong political leadership and genuine commitment, without which the most well designed and appropriate programmes are likely to founder. Countries such as Thailand, Brazil, Uganda, and Senegal have seen a dramatic impact on their rates of STIs and HIV, which has been facilitated greatly by political support at the highest level.

Interventions that reduce the rate of STI can be aimed at the entire community or targeted at specific groups who are at high risk of, or are particularly vulnerable to, infection. One to one prevention interventions can take place in clinic settings, as outlined in Chapter 3.

Primary prevention

Primary prevention interventions aim to keep people uninfected. These approaches are obviously not mutually

---

Determinants of STI spread

$$R_0 = \beta cd$$

R_0 = average number of new infections that result from one infection

β = transmissibility

c = average rate of acquiring partners

d = duration of infection

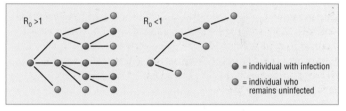

Pattern of spread

Principles of effective STI control

- Reduce infectiousness of STIs
  - Condoms
- Reduce duration of infection
  - Encourage diagnosis and treatment of symptomatic infection (encourage health seeking behaviour) and asymptomatic infection (screening, partner notification, and mass or targeted treatment)
- Reduce risky behaviour
  - Reduce rate of partner change
  - Delay onset of sexual intercourse
  - Improve selection of partners

Primary prevention

- *Behavioural interventions* are aimed at enhancing knowledge, skills, and attitudes to help people protect themselves against infection (for example, health promotion to decrease partner change and increase condom use)
- *Structural interventions* are aimed at broader societal and economic issues that drive the spread of STIs
- *Biomedical interventions* include condoms, vaccines, vaginal microbicides, or male circumcision to prevent the acquisition of infection

exclusive. Individual behaviour change probably will be best sustained in a community that is broadly supportive. In addition, the broader cultural mores of the community will influence greatly the feasibility of delivering education in that community and will also affect how people respond to it.

Education and information

The aim of sexual health promotion is broader than minimising the risks associated with sexual intercourse and other sexual practices. It also aims to facilitate development of healthy sexual behaviour patterns and relationships. Although supplying appropriate and timely factual information is very important and the first step in this process, evidence shows that providing information alone is not enough to bring about a change in behaviour. Widely available information about STIs (or contraception) has not been proved to encourage immoral or promiscuous behaviour.

Health education needs to inform people of the advantages of discriminate and safer sex and the means to prevent or reduce the risk of infection. Although the best way to avoid STIs is to avoid sexual intercourse, this is not a realistic or acceptable message. People need health messages that are tailored to their lifestyles and needs, which allow them to make informed choices about their behaviour. Factors other than lack of knowledge contribute to an individual's ability to practice safer sexual behaviour, however, including perception of health risk, low self esteem, poor self efficacy, peer pressure, and power and sex inequalities. Drug and alcohol use also have an influence. Increasingly, health promotion interventions aim to address some or all of these factors.

That health promotion campaigns address the issues directly related to the infections themselves is also important, including what the various infections are; how to recognise the symptoms; the short and long term consequences of infection; and where to access appropriate advice, diagnosis, and treatment. As most of those infected with an STI have either asymptomatic or unrecognised infection, however, people also need to be aware that they cannot rely on symptoms alone to distinguish infected people from uninfected people and that they themselves can be infected even if asymptomatic.

Structural or societal interventions

Clearly it may be unrealistic to expect individual behaviour change when the broader societal and cultural context is not supportive of this change.

Structural factors that may hinder behaviour change include physical, social, cultural, organisational, economic, and legal or policy aspects of the environment. For example, interventions that promote condom use and partner reduction strategies for impoverished heterosexual women in developing countries may be impractical, because women lack the power to negotiate condom use, particularly with their regular partners or husbands, and because they may be economically dependent on sex work to provide income for basic necessities, such as food or their children's school fees. In this scenario, interventions need to include men and, more broadly, tackle women's rights regarding inheritance, owning property, and earning income legitimately.

Biomedical interventions

Male condoms, if used properly and consistently, can reduce the risk of transmission of many STIs. They are more effective for some STIs than for others, however, and their use does not guarantee that infection will not occur. Female condoms are also advocated to reduce STI and HIV transmission and are attractive because they are under the control of the woman,

Ways for an individual to reduce their risk of contracting an STI

- Abstain
- Have a mutually monogamous relationship with someone who is uninfected
- Select partners whose past and current behaviour puts them at low risk of infection. Consider both being screened for infection before unprotected sex
- Reduce the numbers of sexual partners
- Avoid sex with people who have symptoms of a STI or oral "cold sores"
- Use condoms consistently on every occasion with all partners
- In open relationships couples agree to have only non-penetrative or protected sex outside their main relationship

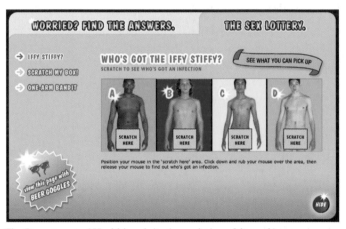

The Department of Health's website (www.playingsafely.co.uk) uses interactive quizzes to show the difficulty in distinguishing infected from uninfected people

Interventions that are most effective are those that draw on social and psychological theories of behaviour change derived from research that seeks to understand the origins and control of sexual behaviour

Structural interventions

These can take place at various levels, including

- Community level (for example, legislating to change the age of consent for homosexual men or inheritance laws)
- Organisational level (for example, providing reproductive health clinics in schools or the workplace)
- Individual level (for example, microfinance initiatives that seek to train women to become less economically dependent)

although evidence of their effectiveness is less than for the male condom.

Hepatitis B vaccine is the only vaccine that effectively prevents acquisition of an STI, although vaccines for other STIs are currently in development or being evaluated. In addition, several other biomedical approaches for reducing the risk of STIs are currently being explored, including presumptive periodic treatment for people who are at high risk of STIs, male circumcision, and vaginal microbicides. However, all these interventions are in the early stages of evaluation.

Secondary prevention

Secondary prevention interventions aim to reduce the risk of individuals infected with an STI transmitting this infection to their sexual partners. These approaches entail increasing screening and appropriate treatment of symptomatic and asymptomatic people; encouraging health seeking behaviour; and tracing, screening, and treating sexual partners of infected people (contact tracing). Other more experimental approaches have included presumptive treatment of people at high risk of infection.

Screening and treatment
Early diagnosis and treatment are cheap, whereas the late sequelae of untreated disease are expensive. For example, if gonorrhoea and chlamydial infection (a major cause of pelvic inflammatory disease (PID)) are well controlled, then PID and all its serious long term sequelae can be prevented.

In many parts of the world specialised STI clinics have been established to provide screening and treatment for people with symptoms of, or who feel they are at risk of, an STI. These clinics provide prompt laboratory or microbiological based diagnosis (or both) and treatment, minimise the incidence of complications and disability, trace and treat sexual contacts, and provide education. These are sometimes known as vertical services.

Clearly the extent of screening will vary according to the laboratory facilities available. In most western countries, clinics screen for syphilis, gonorrhoea, chlamydia, *Trichomonas vaginalis*, bacterial vaginosis, and *Candida* as a matter of course and offer HIV antibody testing. Those presenting with symptoms will have additional screening tests (see Chapters 3-7). Screening at an STI clinic, however, does not guarantee that a person is free of all infections. It is not routine to screen asymptomatic individuals for herpes simplex virus or human papillomavirus. Those people found to be infected should be managed according to local treatment guidelines. Increasingly, single dose treatments are available for STIs, and the use of these will maximise compliance and minimise the development of drug resistance.

In countries without access to a laboratory, most people who present to clinic will be symptomatic, and screening may be limited to clinical examination with or without microscopy. The sensitivity and specificity of clinical examination for distinguishing STI causes of genital symptoms from non-STI causes, particularly in women, has improved somewhat by using a system for scoring risk. For example, having had a new partner recently greatly increases an person's risk of contracting an STI. The services are non-specialised and provided as part of other general medical services, for example in primary health centres, maternal and child health centres, and family planning clinics, and by private practitioners, pharmacists, traditional healers, and street

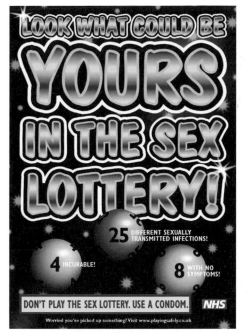

The Department of Health's website (www.playingsafely.co.uk) promotes the use of condoms for sexual health

---

Secondary prevention
- Enhancing health seeking behaviour
- Improving access to for STIs diagnosis and treatment
- Ensuring appropriate case management
- Early detection and treatment of symptomatic and asymptomatic infection
- Partner notification (contact tracing)

To be most effective, clinics should be open access and provide confidential, non-judgmental care and appropriate health care for which there is no charge. Health education can be used to enhance health seeking behaviour and to encourage people without symptoms to attend for screening if they are at high risk of infection

---

Specialist services for STIs in the United Kingdom
- Genitourinary medicine—269 clinics and 273 consultants
- Features of service
  - Open access and free
  - Confidential
  - Screening and treatment for STIs
  - Screening and treatment for HIV
  - Contraception and psychosexual problems
  - Miscellaneous care (for example, for urinary tract infections and genital dermatological conditions)
  - Partner notification
  - Health promotion, counselling, and advice
  - Outreach and special services
  - Training and research

vendors. Vertical and integrated services for managing individuals with STIs have both advantages and disadvantages.

In resource poor settings where clinics have limited access to diagnostic facilities, the World Health Organization recommends that the syndromic approach is used for patient management. This uses algorithms based on the common presenting signs and symptoms, for example genital ulceration and urethral or vaginal discharge. Rather than healthcare worker trying to decide on the aetiology of the symptoms on the basis of examination alone, the relevant algorithm shows treatment for all the common STI causes of that syndrome in that setting. Syndromic management algorithms differ in different parts of the world, which reflects the local disease profile and antimicrobial resistance patterns (examples are given in Chapters 5 and 7). In some countries where much of the treatment for STIs is delivered through pharmacists and street vendors, preprepared drug treatment packages have been developed and marketed. These packs include the appropriate drug for the relevant syndrome, a contact slip advising that the sexual partner should be treated, and will often include condoms as well.

In addition to managing people who present with symptoms, the syndromic approach has been supplemented in some settings by presumptively treating people who are at high risk of bacterial STIs with appropriate antibiotics. For example, in South Africa, a programme that provides monthly antibiotic treatment to sex workers seems to have reduced the rates of bacterial STIs among sex workers and their clients. This approach is attractive because it allows treatment of symptomatic and asymptomatic people, although it needs to be evaluated more formally to see if it results in the development of antimicrobial resistance or any other adverse effects. An extension of this is the concept of mass treatment of whole populations who have or might be at risk of STIs.

Contact tracing

Tracing sexual contacts is an important part of any control programme. Sexual contacts have an increased likelihood of infection with an STI and are often (although not always) unaware that they are infected. It is essential, therefore, to get in touch with contacts as soon as possible and advise them to attend a clinic. Although contact tracing is primarily conducted for its public health benefit, it also is of direct benefit to the people concerned. For someone in an ongoing relationship, treatment of their partner is essential if they are not to become reinfected. If the contact remains unaware of their infection risk, they may go on to develop sequelae of infection or to infect other people unwittingly.

Vertical services for STIs

Advantages	Disadvantages
• Specialists	• Expensive
• Accurate laboratory diagnosis with appropriate treatment	• Delays in diagnosis
	• Limited availability
• Reference laboratory	• Limited coverage of population
• Training	• Stigmatisation
• Monitoring, surveillance, and research	• Poor sustainability
• Asymptomatic infection may be detected	

Integrated services for STIs

Advantages	Disadvantages
• Problem orientated	• Low sensitivity and specificity for cervical gonococcal or chlamydial infection in women
• Immediate presumptive diagnosis and treatment of possible aetiologies	
• Non-specialist	• Asymptomatic infection not detected but treatment possible by active partner notification and epidemiological treatment of partners
• Inexpensive	
• Standardisation of management and monitoring of drug use and antibiotic resistance	• Not always acceptable to medical staff

---

Contact tracing

- *Patient (index) referral*, whereby the patient informs their sexual partners themselves
- *Provider referral*, whereby the index patient asks the healthcare worker to inform partners on their behalf
- *Contract (conditional) referral*, whereby the index patient undertakes to notify partners themselves in a given timeframe. If the partners are not notified in this period, the contact tracer or health adviser will attempt to notify them with the patient's consent. This uses a combination of the patient and provider referral techniques

---

Further reading

- Mathews C, Coaetzee N, Zwarenstein M, Lombard C, Guttmacher S. Strategies for partner notification for sexually transmitted diseases. *Cochrane Database Syst Rev* 2004;(1):CD002843
- Sumartojo E, Doll L, Holtgrave D, Gayle H, Merson M. Enriching the mix: incorporating structural factors into HIV prevention. *AIDS* 2000;14:S1-2
- Evidence of effectiveness of HIV prevention interventions. *JAIDS* 2002;30:S1-134
- Holmes KK. Human ecology and behaviour and sexually transmitted bacterial infections. *Proc Nat Acad Sci* 1994;91:2448-55
- Parker R, Easton D, Klein C. Structural barriers and facilitators in HIV prevention: a review of international research. *AIDS* 2000;4:22-3

3 The clinical process

Patrick French

People with sexually transmitted infections (STIs) are often asymptomatic or have symptoms that they do not recognise as being related to an STI. They also may not have access to care or be unaware of how to access care. They can be identified in many ways, however, in a wide range of differing services and settings. The most appropriate site for STI care will reflect local epidemiology, the resources available for care, and the pre-existing structure of health services. This will mean that, according to local circumstances, STI care could be provided by primary or secondary care, pharmacies, or outreach services (see Chapter 2). In the United Kingdom, STIs often are managed by specialists in genitourinary medicine in dedicated clinics.

Despite the need for clinical services to reflect diversity, it is also important to ensure that some key principles regarding the care of people with STIs are adopted. They should receive effective treatment and care as promptly as possible. This approach reduces the risk of the patient developing complications and reduces the chances of onward transmission.

Facilitation of the access of people with STIs or at risk of STIs to services that provide assessment and care is an essential step in establishing good control of STIs. Linking services to any health promotion activity in the community that is designed to raise awareness of STIs and establishing care pathways with other non-specialist clinical services are all part of this access strategy.

Another vital component is service advertising. The media used for advertising will depend on the target populations of the local STI programme and the resources available.

Services for people who seek care for STIs should encourage destigmatisation of these conditions and also acknowledge that such stigma exists. Establishing an environment that is confidential, private, and free of judgment encourages openness and allows a full and accurate risk assessment to be undertaken. This lays the groundwork for future care and health promotion.

Care of individuals with STIs often requires the participation of a multidisciplinary team of practitioners including nurses, doctors, administration staff, laboratory workers, and counsellors. Staff who are responsible for helping to identify and trace sexual contacts are an essential part of the team. In the United Kingdom, this work often is undertaken by sexual health advisers. The effectiveness of the team is enhanced greatly by shared clinical guidelines and operational

---

Summary of the clinical process

- Presentation to STI service
- Sexual history and risk assessment
- Clinical and genital examination
- Investigations
- Treatment
- Condoms
- Health promotion
- Partner management
- Follow up

Ways STIs can be identified

- Screening
- Case finding ("opportunistic" screening)
- Presentation to non-STI clinical services
- Presentation (including self referral) to STI services

Principles of STI care

- Access to care must be easy, rapid, and preferably free
- Systematic risk assessment of all patients is needed
- Investigations should support but not delay care
- Rapid and "bedside" tests are important
- Therapy that is easy to adhere is preferable (single dose if possible)
- Condom and sexual health promotion
- Partner management

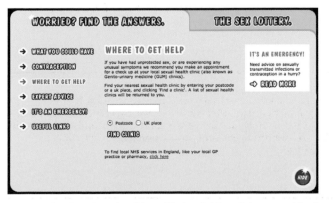

An example of service advertising—Playing Safely website created by the Department of Health, United Kingdom (www.playingsafely.co.uk)

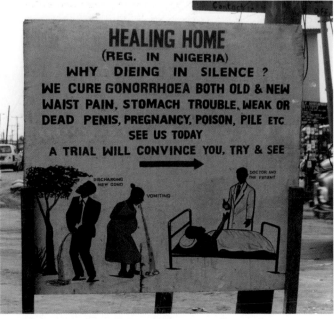

An example of service advertising—STI care in the developing world

policies, which include a description of the roles and responsibilities of each staff group.

Core components of STI assessment

The core components of an STI assessment are history taking (especially sexual history), examination (particularly genital examination), and investigations.

Sexual history taking

The communication skills required to take a good sexual history are an extension of the skills already possessed by many healthcare workers. It is important to establish rapport and trust between the doctor and patient and to acknowledge that many people find it difficult to discuss their sexual lives openly.

The scope and detail of the sexual history will vary according to the site of care, available resources (particularly consultation time), and the particular patient group being seen. However, to allow for basic risk assessment and further management several crucial components must be discussed. The specific issues that relate to sexual history taking in men and women are detailed in Chapters 5 and 7, respectively.

The sexual history will guide the clinical examination and will allow for a more rational approach to selecting investigations. The sexual history will also form the basis for partner management and sexual health promotion. The period of time over which a sexual history should look back will depend on a number of factors, including duration of symptoms (if any symptoms are present), the date of previous STI assessments, and incubation periods of any STIs diagnosed or suspected. In practice, most clinicians would elicit a risk history for at least the previous three months or until the last partner change, whichever is the longer. Ideally, the sexual history should form part of a wider risk history that should include a general medical history, including current drug use and misuse (including injecting drug use) and allergies. In women cervical cytology, gynaecology, and contraception histories should be taken. For proformas see Appendix on pages 85–6.

Clinical examination

The clinical examination is an important part of the assessment for an STI and will be guided by the sexual history. Often during the examination, clinical specimens are obtained and some STIs are diagnosed. Sexually transmissible conditions, such as scabies, pediculosis pubis, molluscum contagiosum, and genital warts, are almost always diagnosed clinically; diagnostic procedures are reserved for atypical presentations.

An appropriate environment for an examination is important. It is essential to explain and discuss the purpose and nature of the examination to the patient and to acknowledge that many patients find it distressing and intrusive. Good visualisation of the genital area is vital for a proper examination. However, the autonomy and dignity of the patient must be recognised and protected as much as possible.

Investigations

The role of the laboratory is discussed in detail in Chapter 17, and sampling during the clinical examination is discussed in Chapter 4.

Diagnostic tests often are taken during the clinical examination but increasingly "non-invasive" tests (including vaginal and vulval tests), in which urine or saliva specimens taken by the patient, are used for diagnosis. Because non-invasive tests are easy to take and samples can be obtained from patients at venues with minimal clinical facilities, they are

> Good management of STIs is not complex but does include a number of important components that need to be addressed during clinical care. For this reason many units have developed proformas to ensure that a systematic and comprehensive approach to management is followed. Such forms also facilitate the routine auditing and improvement of clinical practice

Sexual history taking

- Symptoms (including duration)
- Last sexual intercourse
- Sex of partner
- Relationship with partner (casual, long term, traceable, etc)
- Use of barrier contraception
- Sites of exposure (oral, vaginal, or anal)
- Last previous partner or partner change (with site of exposure and barrier contraception history as above)
- Partners' symptoms
- Previous STIs or testing for STIs including HIV

Name:	Date:
Sex:	Number:
Age:	Scen by:
Status:	
Main symptom:	Sexual History:
Previous STI:	Examination findings:
Condom knowledge: Condom use:	
Treatment received so far:	
Drug allergy:	
Diagnosis:	Treatment:
Counselling: Compliance Contacts Condoms STI/HIV prevention	Signature:
Follow up:	

Developing world proforma: a case record can be designed on one page to record essential information about STI patients

Examination setting

- Clear explanation to patient
- Comfortable for patient and clinician
- Private
- Good illumination
- Chaperoning for patient

> The diagnostic investigations undertaken will depend on the findings during risk assessment and clinical examination, as well as the resources available to the doctor

particularly well suited to screening and case finding programmes.

In some settings, the most effective form of STI care and control is syndromic management (see Chapters 5, 7, 8, and 11), so that no investigations are taken to establish an aetiological diagnosis. This approach will usually include the components described earlier and health promotion and partner management, but treatment is administered according to local knowledge of the cause or aetiology of the presenting syndrome (such as treating men presenting with urethral discharge for gonorrhoea and chlamydia).

In other environments, rapid and bedside investigations aid diagnosis during the initial clinic visit. These are particularly useful in the rapid diagnosis of urethral gonorrhoea in men and determining the aetiology of vaginal discharge. The range of tests currently undertaken in STI clinics in the United Kingdom is discussed in Chapters 4-7.

Treatment of STIs

Treatments for STIs need to be effective and administered as promptly as possible. A relatively small number of drugs are needed to provide effective therapy for most of the infections, and this allows many services to develop small onsite dispensaries.

National and international guidelines for STI treatment have been developed to improve and standardise care. They are evidence based and updated on a regular basis. With the exceptions of gonorrhoea and chancroid, little clinically important resistance to the recommended antimicrobials is seen. An effective single dose treatment is now available for most bacterial and protozoal STIs, including gonorrhoea, chlamydia, syphilis, chancroid, and trichomoniasis. This allows onsite observed therapy and removes concerns about treatment adherence.

Treatment for viral STIs is more complex and will often require long term follow up and care. The role of treatment in reducing the infectiousness of viral STIs is being elucidated at present, but it is probable that sexual health promotion and condom promotion have equally important roles.

The dosing schedule, rationale, and possible toxicities must be discussed with the patient, as well as potential interactions with other therapies, for example antibiotics and oral contraceptives.

Condom and sexual health promotion

A consultation with patients who have STIs or are at risk of developing an STI is a valuable opportunity to provide sexual health promotion, prevention, education, and condom promotion on a one to one basis.

The areas covered in a sexual health promotion discussion will be similar in all consultations but can be tailored to the needs of the individual patient. Hepatitis A and B are currently the only STIs that can be prevented by vaccination (herpes simplex type II infection and HPV-16 vaccines are being developed).

Many STI services and prevention programmes offer hepatitis B vaccination to all STI patients or to some who are perceived as being at particularly high risk of acquiring hepatitis B (see Chapter 15).

People with STIs or attending STI services are much more likely than the general population to have HIV infection. Offering and recommending HIV testing should be a routine part of all STI consultations

---

Treatment guidelines*

- Clinical effectiveness produced by the British Association for Sexual Health and HIV (UK) 2002 (www.bashh.org)
- International Union against STIs (European) 2001 (www.iusti.org)
- Centers for Disease Control (American) 2002 (www.cdc.gov/cdc/std/treatment/SumCont.htm)
- World Health Organization 2002 (www.who.int/docstore/hiv/STIManagemntguidelines/)

*All treatment recommendations cited in the text are taken from one or more of the guidelines above

---

Treatment of STIs

Features of effective therapy

- Prompt administration
- Observed therapy or single dose treatment
- Well tolerated or easy adherence
- Guidelines followed (local gonorrhoea or chancroid sensitivities)

Treatment discussion

- Nature or rationale of therapy
- Written information
- Treatment adherence
- Sexual abstinence during treatment
- Partner notification
- Follow up (if needed)

Sexual health promotion

- Behaviour change
- Safer sex and risk reduction
- Condom promotion
- Hepatitis B vaccination
- Future STI care

Partner management

All patients with STIs will have had at least one partner who currently has or who has previously had an infection. Partner notification is an essential part of care (see Chapter 2). Encouraging the sexual partners of patients with an STI to attend for assessment, treatment, and care reduces the risk of reinfection of the index patient, allows identification of STIs in individuals who are asymptomatic or who have unrecognised symptoms, and provides an opportunity to discuss sexual health promotion with someone at high risk of an STI.

Partner notification entails a sensitive discussion that relies on establishing trust between the patient and healthcare worker. The rationale and importance of partner notification should be explained clearly to the patient. Most patients will take on the responsibility of informing their sexual contacts (patient referral), but some patients may request or need the clinic to undertake partner notification on their behalf (provider referral).

Contact slips and written information for patients and their sexual contacts may facilitate this process. Mechanisms for monitoring the outcome of partner management should be established.

Follow up

Many patients with infections will need follow up care. This may be related to directly reviewing the outcome of previous treatment and the management of viral STIs. However, it may also include testing for STIs with long incubation periods (such as HIV and syphilis) and further health promotion activity.

It is essential that follow up appointments check for

- Symptom resolution
- Treatment adherence
- Further sexual exposure
- Partner notification resolution
- Test of cure or treatment response
- Further STI screening
- Health promotion.

MORTIMER MARKET CENTRE
Mortimer Market
London, WC1E 6AU

Tel: 020 7530 5050

Open:
Mon	9.00a.m. - 6.00p.m.	
Tues	9.00a.m. - 11.00a.m.	
	3.45p.m. - 7.00p.m.	
Wed	9.00a.m. - 6.00p.m.	
Thurs	9.00a.m. - 6.00p.m.	
fri	9.00a.m. - 2.45p.m.	

On receipt of this slip we strongly advise you to make an appointment as soon as possible by ringing 020 7530 5050, Monday - Friday.

If you would like to speak to a health professional, in confidence, about this slip please ring 020 7530 5111.

This is a free and confidential service.

PLEASE BRING THIS SLIP WITH YOU WHEN YOU ATTEND AND GIVE TO THE DOCTOR

FOR CLINIC USE ONLY

INDEX REF NO: CONTACT REF NO......

DATE: DATE: ...

KC60 CODE: KC60 CODE:

PLEASE RETURN TO HEALTH ADVISERS DEPARTMENT, MORTIMER MARKET CENTRE

Contact slip

The developing world proforma is adapted from *Providing Health Services in Sexual Health Interventions*. West Bengal: Project Management Unit of the West Bengal Sexual Health Project, 1998.

4 Examination techniques and clinical sampling

Patrick French

The general principles and appropriate environment for the examination were covered in Chapter 3. In practice, the examination of patients in a clinic is often confined to the genitals, but if a sexually transmitted infection (STI) that has extragenital manifestations is suspected (such as scabies, syphilis, or HIV), then a general examination will also be necessary, even if the patient has no symptoms outside the genitalia. This examination will concentrate on the skin, mouth, and lymph nodes but a more thorough examination is essential if the late complications of HIV or syphilis are suspected.

Examination of the male patient

Examination of the male genitalia may be done standing (useful for hernia and varicocoele) or lying. It should include

- inspection of areas covered with hair for pediculosis pubis
- examination of genital skin for ulceration, inflammation, warts, and molluscum contagiosum
- palpation of inguinal lymph nodes for enlargement and tenderness
- retraction of the prepuce and a search for subpreputial skin lesions (such as chancre or warts) and balanitis
- urethral meatus for discharge and meatitis (the patient or doctor may try to squeeze out the discharge)
- palpation of the testes and epididymes to diagnose epididymo-orchitis and screen for testicular cancer.

The anus should be inspected externally for warts that occur in both homosexual and heterosexual males. Men who report anal symptoms, receptive anal intercourse, or receptive oroanal sexual contact should undergo proctoscopy to inspect the anal and rectal mucosa for inflammation, pus, or ulcers. Digital examination may assist in diagnosing prostatic disorders, such as cancer and prostatic inflammation.

As previously mentioned, clinical sampling often will be taken during examination, and the routine tests taken are described below. Other tests will be dictated by clinical presentation and local epidemiology. All patients should be offered and recommended serological tests for syphilis and HIV (after pre-test discussion).

Sampling of the male patient

Urethra
A plastic loop is inserted to a depth of 2 cm and smeared on to a glass slide for Gram staining and enumeration of polymorphs to diagnose urethritis. It can then be streaked on to gonococcal culture medium. A second specimen is taken for chlamydia testing.

Urine
All tests listed above can also be done on a spun urine deposit. Some services use leucocyte esterase testing to indicate a possible diagnosis of urethritis.

Throat (if indicated)
A Dacron tipped swab is taken from the tonsillar crypts and posterior pharynx and plated on to gonococcal culture medium. Gram stained smears from this site are not helpful.

General examination

Skin
- Scabies—rash (especially on wrists, between the fingers, and on as the buttocks and areolae)
- Secondary syphilis and HIV (seroconversion illness)—generalised rash and lesions on palms and soles

Lymph nodes
- Secondary syphilis, HIV, and primary herpes simplex—generalised lymphadenopathy

Mouth
- Secondary syphilis—ulceration and mucous patches
- HIV—oral hairy leukoplakia, oral candidiasis, Kaposi's sarcoma, and angular cheilosis
- Herpes simplex—ulceration
- Warts

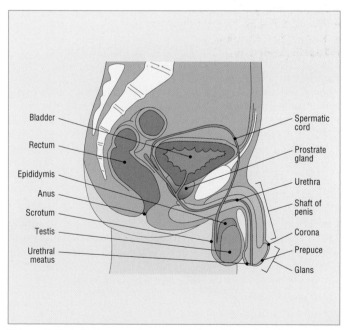

Male genitalia including scrotal contents (adapted from *Sexually transmitted infections: history taking and examination* CD, The Wellcome Trust, 2003)

Rectum (if indicated)

The rectal mucosa is sampled through a proctoscope with a plastic loop that is smeared on to a glass slide for Gram staining and streaked on to gonococcal culture medium.

Prostate (if indicated)

Sampling prostatic fluid requires firm massage of the prostate gland with a gloved finger inserted in the rectum to express prostatic secretions through to the urethral meatus. Material obtained can then be examined in stained smears and cultured.

Examination of the female patient

Examination of the female patient begins with an inspection of the external genitalia, followed by vaginal and cervical examination after passing a vaginal speculum (usually a Cusco speculum). Finally, a bimanual pelvic examination is done.

External genitalia

- Examine genital skin for inflammation, ulcers, warts, molluscum contagiosum, and pediculosis pubis
- Examine vestibule and introitus for any discharge or Bartholin's cyst or abscess
- Palpate inguinal lymph nodes.

Cervix and vagina

- Inspect discharge
- Examine vaginal walls for inflammation
- Examine cervix for ectropion, cervicitis, and mucopurulent discharge.

Pelvis

- Examine uterus and cervix for pain on palpation or movement
- Examine for adnexal tenderness and masses.

Sampling of the female patient

Vagina

Vaginal discharge samples are taken from the posterior fornix with a small plastic loop. The discharge is tested with narrow range pH paper and potassium hydroxide to help elucidate the cause of the vaginal discharge.

A further vaginal sample is examined in wet preparation for *Trichomonas vaginalis* and clue cells and with gram stain for *Candida albicans*. The vaginal sample is sent for *T vaginalis* and *C albicans* culture.

Cervix

After mucus and secretions have been wiped off the cervix with a cotton wool ball, the endocervix is sampled. A loop is used to take a sample for Gram staining and *Neisseria gonorrhoeae* culture. A further swab is taken for the identification of *Chlamydia trachomatis*.

Urethra

A small plastic loop is used to collect a sample from the proximal urethra that is smeared on to a glass slide for Gram staining and streaked on to a slide for *N gonorrhoeae* culture.

A full description of laboratory diagnostic tests used in the field of STIs is given in Chapter 17.

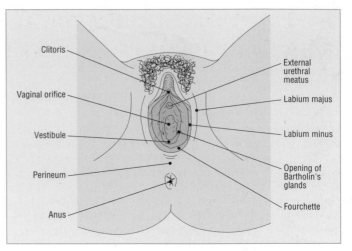

Female external genitalia (adapted from *Sexually transmitted infections: history taking and examination* CD, The Wellcome Trust, 2003)

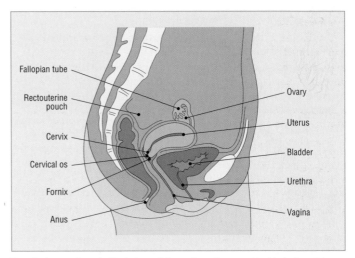

Female internal genitalia (adapted from *Sexually transmitted infections: history taking and examination* CD, The Wellcome Trust, 2003)

Proctoscopy and tests for *N gonorrhoeae* should be done for all women who report anal sex

5 Main presentations of sexually transmitted infections in male patients

John Richens

Some sexually transmitted infections (STIs), such as gonorrhoea and chlamydial infection, have very different presentations in the two sexes because of differences in genital anatomy. This chapter focuses on infections of the male urethra, epididymis, testis, and prostate. Anal and oral symptoms are also covered because these are encountered more often among men, especially men who have sex with men. Chapter 6 deals with a variety of other genital symptoms in men that usually are not related to STIs but often come to the attention of healthcare professionals who work in sexual health services.

Urethral discharge and dysuria

Spontaneous discharge of fluid from the urethral meatus, usually most noticeable after holding the urine overnight and often accompanied by burning discomfort during urination (dysuria), strongly indicates a sexually acquired urethral infection.

Symptomatic gonorrhoea usually develops in a few days of exposure. *Chlamydia* infections take slightly longer. Mild infections may cause urethral discomfort and dysuria without discharge and may be confused with cystitis.

Management of urethritis in male patients

1 Take history, including sexual history
2 Examine, looking especially for evidence of discharge
3 Take samples from urethra
4 Treat for gonorrhoea and chlamydia if urethral Gram stain is positive for Gram negative intracellular diplococci
5 Give treatment for *Chlamydia* if the urethral smear shows five or more polymorphs per high power field and the Gram stain does not suggest gonorrhoea
6 Explain diagnosis, treatment, and methods of prevention
7 Advise to avoid sex until treatment and follow up are completed
8 Advise partner treatment
9 Review patient after treatment for symptoms, adherence, treatment of partners, and test of cure if gonorrhoea has been diagnosed

Where laboratory investigation is not feasible, steps 3, 5, and the test of cure can be omitted

Causes of urethritis in men

Common diagnoses among men with urethritis

- Gonorrhoea
- Chlamydial infection
- Non-specific urethritis

Less common diagnoses among men with urethritis

- *Ureaplasma urealyticum* infection
- *Mycoplasma genitalium* infection
- Trichomoniasis
- Herpes simplex virus infection
- *Escherichia coli* infection
- Bacteroides infection
- Cystitis
- Pyelonephritis
- Trauma
- Foreign body
- Reactive arthritis, Reiter's syndrome, and allied conditions

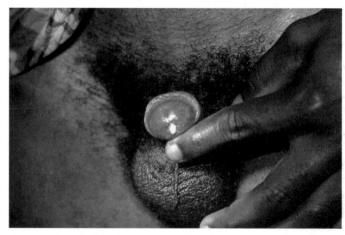

Gonococcal urethral discharge

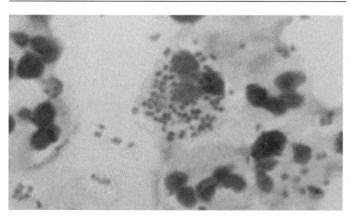

Gram negative intracellular diplococci

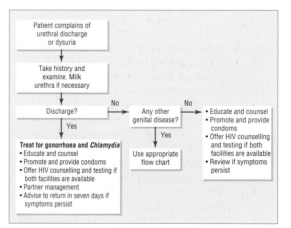

Urethral discharge flow chart (World Health Organization)

Overview of chlamydial and gonorrhoea infection

Chlamydia

Cause
- *Chlamydia trachomatis*, types D-K (see also lymphogranuloma venereum, p 45). *C trachomatis* is an obligate intracellular bacterium

Initial sites of infection
- Epithelial cells of urethra, cervix, rectum, pharynx, and conjunctiva depending on mode of exposure

Incubation period
- Less than four weeks for men; unknown in women
- Asymptomatic infections are common in both sexes and can persist for many months

Main symptoms in men
- Urethral discharge and dysuria

Less common symptoms in men
- Proctitis, conjunctivitis, epididymo-orchitis, and reactive arthritis

Main symptoms in women
- Dysuria, vaginal discharge, and intermenstrual bleeding

Less common symptoms in women
- Pelvic inflammatory disease (with sequelae of infertility and ectopic pregnancy), perihepatitis (Fitz-Hugh-Curtis syndrome), and conjunctivitis

Symptoms affecting neonates
- Conjunctivitis and pneumonia

Main methods of diagnosis
- Enzyme immunoassay and DNA amplification (ligase chain reaction (LCR) and polymerase chain reaction) (see Chapter 17)

Recommended treatments for uncomplicated Chlamydia
- Doxycyline: 100 mg twice daily for seven days (C, E, U, W)
- Azithromycin: 1 g single dose (C, E, U, W)
- Erythromycin base: 500 mg twice daily for 14 days (E (2), U(2))
- Erythromycin base: 500 mg four times daily for seven days (C (2), E(2), U(2), W)
- Erythromycin ethylsuccinate: 800 mg four times daily for seven days (C(2))
- Tetracycline: 500 mg four times daily for seven days (U(2), W)
- Ofloxacin: 200-300 mg twice daily or 400 mg once daily for seven days (C(2), E(2), U(2), W)
- Levofloxacin: 500 mg daily for seven days (C)
- Amoxicillin: 500 mg three times daily for seven days has been validated in pregnant patients (C, E, U, W)

Follow up testing
- Not recommended routinely and should not be done before three weeks if PCR or LCR is used, because these tests can detect non-viable organisms

(C = Centers for Disease Control, USA; E = European STI guidelines; U = UK National Guidelines; W = World Health Organization; (2) = second line recommendation).

Gonorrhoea

Cause
- *Neisseria gonorrhoeae*, a Gram negative coccus
- Initial sites of infection: columnar epithelium of urethra, endocervix, rectum, pharynx, or conjunctiva depending on mode of exposure

Incubation period
- Two to five days in 80% of men who develop urethral symptoms
- Asymptomatic infections common in both sexes, especially infections of pharynx, cervix, and rectum

Main symptoms in men
- Urethral discharge, dysuria, and tender inguinal lymph nodes

Less common genital symptoms in men
- Epididymo-orchitis, abscesses of paraurethral glands, and urethral stricture

Main symptoms in women
- Vaginal discharge, dysuria, abnormal bleeding
- Examination may show mucopurulent discharge from the cervical os, urethra, Skene's glands, or Bartholin's glands

Less common genital symptoms in women
- Lower abdominal pain and vulvovaginitis (pre-pubertal girls)

Extragenital symptoms and complications that affect both sexes
- Pharyngitis, rectal pain and discharge, and conjunctivitis
- Disseminated infection involving skin, joints, and heart valves, secondary infertility after damage to Fallopian tubes, or epididymis

Main methods of diagnosis
- Detection of Gram negative intracellular diplococci in smears and culture for *N gonorrhoeae*

Treatments recommended for uncomplicated gonorrhoea in the following guidelines
- Ciprofloxacin: 500 mg single dose by mouth (C, E, U, W)
- Ofloxacin: 400 mg single dose by mouth (C, E, U, W)
- Levofloxacin: 250 mg single dose by mouth (C)
- Ceftriaxone: 125 mg single dose given intramuscularly (C, E, U(2), W)
- Cefotaxime: 500 mg single dose given intramuscularly (C(2), U(2))
- Cefixime: 400 mg single dose given by mouth (C, E, W)
- Spectinomycin: 2 g single dose given intramuscularly (C(2), E, U(2), W)
- Ampicillin: 2 g or 3 g plus probenecid 1 g as a single oral dose (U, E(2)) (in areas with <5% resistance to penicillin)

Resistance
- Resistance to penicillin and tetracyclines is widespread Resistance to quinolones is increasing and resistance to azithromycin and spectinomycin has been reported
- Choice of treatment should take into account local susceptibility data

Follow up
- A test of cure culture is recommended when available

In clinics with laboratory facilities, the usual approach is to test for gonorrhoea and chlamydial infection. The first step is microscopy of a urethral smear. Optimal results for this are obtained from patients who have held their urine for four hours or more.

Urethritis is confirmed if the urethral smear shows five or more polymorphs per high power field. If the smear shows Gram negative intracellular diplococci, the patient is treated for gonorrhoea and *Chlamydia* to cover the possibility of a mixed infection. Meanwhile, confirmatory tests for gonorrhoea and *Chlamydia* are carried out (see Chapter 17).

Patients without evidence of gonorrhoea receive doxycycline (100 mg twice daily for one week), erythromycin (500 mg twice daily for two weeks), or azithromycin (1 g single

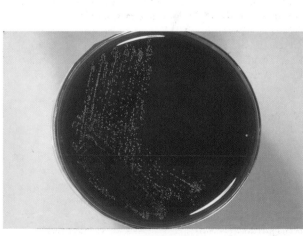

N gonorrhoeae culture

dose), which are active against chlamydial infection and most other pathogens associated with non-gonococcal urethritis. Doxycycline can cause photosensitivity. Absorption is impaired by antacids, iron, calcium, and magnesium salts. Gastrointestinal upset is common with erythromycin and azithromycin.

This approach will relieve symptoms in most patients, but some will report persistent symptoms or show a persistently abnormal smear without symptoms. The options are then to investigate for treatment failure or reinfection or for infection by less common pathogens (for example, *Trichomonas vaginalis*) and to repeat, continue, or change the antibiotic therapy or await spontaneous resolution of symptoms.

When access to laboratory testing is not available, the simplest approach to managing urethritis is to administer blind treatment for gonorrhoea and *Chlamydia*.

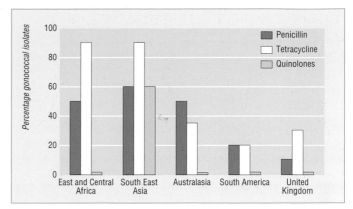

Antimicrobial resistance of *N gonorrhoeae* in selected countries in the 1990s

Scrotal swelling and pain

Mild testicular discomfort in the absence of abnormal physical signs is encountered commonly in young male attenders in STI clinics. Many such patients can be reassured if testicular examination and a screen for STIs are carried out and found to be normal. In some cases, anxiety about infection, sexual function, or cancer is present. More marked scrotal pain has a variety of causes.

Acute inflammation of the scrotal contents (usually unilateral) in young men is usually caused by gonorrhoea or *Chlamydia*. In older men, *Escherichia coli*, klebsiella, pseudomonas, and proteus are found more often. The first consideration in diagnosis is to exclude acute torsion, which requires emergency surgery. Torsion predominates in the teenage years, usually has an acute onset, and is often accompanied by vomiting. An immediate surgical opinion should be sought for any possible case. Doppler scanning is useful for demonstrating impaired blood flow. The distinguishing features of a mumps orchitis are usually onset several days after parotid swelling, severe testicular pain, and marked systemic symptoms, although the parotitis may be absent. Useful tests for cases of suspected epididymo-orchitis are a urethral smear, mid stream urine culture, and investigations for gonorrhoea and chlamydia. Presumptive treatment for gonorrhoea and chlamydia is appropriate in younger males when investigation is not feasible. Severe cases require treatment in hospital with parenteral antibiotics. Analgesia, scrotal support, and elevation may reduce discomfort and promote recovery.

Painless swellings in the scrotum are common. Most of these are small, round, epididymal cysts or spermatocoeles that require no investigation or treatment. Lesions in the testis can be due to tuberculosis, syphilis, or malignancy and require urgent ultrasound examination. Varicocoeles feel like a bag of worms in the scrotum and can be associated with infertility. Therefore, referral to a urologist is advised if pain, testicular atrophy, infertility, or the threat of infertility are concerns.

Pelvic pain in the male

The prostate can be affected by a variety of infectious and poorly defined non-infectious conditions that present as acute or chronic pelvic pain with a range of accompanying urinary and systemic symptoms. Gonorrhoea, chlamydial infections, and trichomoniasis can affect the prostate, but most acute infections are caused by other bacteria such as *E coli*, proteus, *Streptococcus faecalis*, *Klebsiella*, and *Pseudomonas*. STIs and non-sexually transmitted bacterial infections of the prostate

Causes of scrotal swelling and pain in adults and adolescents
- Infections of testis and epididymis: gonorrhoea, *Chlamydia*, tuberculosis, mumps virus, and Gram negative bacteria
- Torsion of testis (mainly adolescents) or appendix testis (mainly three to seven year olds)
- Pain after vasectomy
- Fournier's gangrene
- Vasculitis: Henoch-Schönlein purpura, Kawasaki disease, and Buerger's disease
- Amiodarone therapy
- Tumour
- Hernia
- Trauma

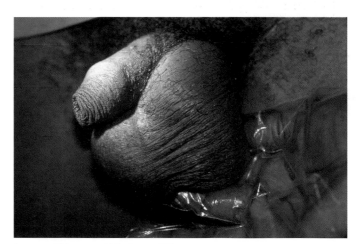

Acute epididymo-orchitis due to STI

Measures occasionally found helpful in men with chronic pelvic pain syndrome
- Simple analgesia
- Non-steroidal anti-inflammatory drugs
- Two to four weeks of ciprofloxacin or doxycycline
- Alpha blocking drugs (alfuzosin, terazosin, tamsulosin)
- Finasteride
- Quercetin
- Low dose amitriptyline
- Repetitive prostatic massage (contraindicated in bacterial prostatitis)
- Regular ejaculation

account for only a few painful prostatic syndromes. Most patients with prostatic pain fall into a category recently designated "chronic pelvic pain syndrome" (CPPS) by the newly adopted National Institutes of Health (NIH) classification of prostatitis syndromes.

In patients who present with pelvic pain, the prostate should be examined for enlargement and tenderness. Patients with prostatitis should undergo a normal screen for STIs. The value of subjecting patients to the unpleasant procedure of prostatic massage to examine prostatic secretions for bacteria and inflammatory cells is now questioned by many experts. Transrectal ultrasonography and urodynamic studies are helpful in some patients. Confirmed infections respond well to antibiotics, the first choice often being a 28 day course of a quinolone or tetracycline, which have better prostatic penetration than other antibiotics.

Treating the more common CPPS is difficult. None of the treatments are well validated, and response rates are often poor. A recently published NIH symptoms index for chronic prostatitis is a useful way to record and monitor symptoms.

Anal symptoms

Anorectal STIs
Sexually transmitted infections can be transmitted by penile-anal contact, oroanal contact, or fingering, resulting in asymptomatic infection, ulceration (for example, herpes and syphilis), warts, or proctitis, the main manifestations of which are pain, tenesmus, bleeding, and discharge. Ulceration is investigated in the same way as genital ulceration (see Chapter 11). Discharges require investigation by proctoscopy, during which samples can be taken from the rectum to test for *Gonorrhoea* and *Chlamydia*. The management of a sexually acquired rectal discharge parallels that of urethritis. Anorectal infections are a potent cofactor for HIV transmission.

Anal intercourse can lead to the transmission of a wide variety of other organisms normally transmitted by the faeco-oral route. These include hepatitis A, *Shigella*, *Salmonella*, and *Giardia*. Anal intraepithelial neoplasia and invasive carcinoma may follow infection with certain subtypes of human papillomavirus.

Non-infectious anal conditions
Patients who practise receptive anal sex often present to STI services with anal fissure, haemorrhoids, perianal haematomas, and pruritus ani. It is important to provide training and guidelines for the management and referral of these common conditions in clinics that see clients who practise anal sex.

Oral and perioral symptoms
Oral STIs usually are asymptomatic. Gonorrhoea and *Chlamydia* infect the pharyngeal mucosa readily but rarely cause acute inflammation. Primary syphilis may present on the tongue or lips, and secondary syphilis can produce an oral mucositis. HIV has an important array of oral manifestations that include oral candidiasis (both erythematous and pseudomembranous), angular cheilitis, gingivitis, oral hairy leucoplakia, and Kaposi's sarcoma. Warts may develop in and around the mouth as a result of orogenital sexual activity.

Differential diagnosis of prostatic pain (NIH classification of prostatitis syndromes)

I	Acute bacterial prostatitis
II	Chronic bacterial prostatitis
III	CPPS
IIIA	CPPS, inflammatory (leucocytes in prostatic secretion, semen, or urine after prostatic massage)
IIIB	CPPS, non-inflammatory (as above without leucocytes)
IV	Asymptomatic inflammatory prostatitis

Other causes of pain in region of prostate
- Pudendal neuralgia (sometimes due to tumour)
- Bladder outlet obstruction
- Bladder tumours
- Urinary stone disease
- Inguinal ligament enthesopathy
- Ejaculatory duct obstruction
- Seminal vesicle calculi
- Bowel disorders

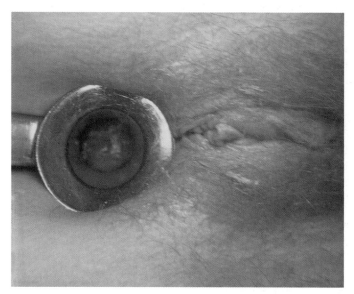

Rectal gonorrhoea

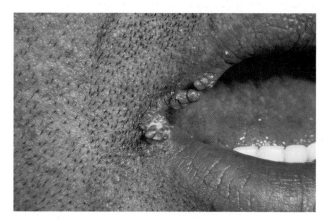

Perioral warts. With permission of the Wellcome Trust

Further reading
- Galejs LE. Diagnosis and treatment of the acute scrotum. *Am Fam Physician* 1999;59:817-24
- Krieger JN, Ross SO, Deutsch L, Riley DE. The NIH Consensus concept of chronic prostatitis/chronic pelvic pain syndrome compared with traditional concepts of nonbacterial prostatitis and prostatodynia. *Curr Urol Rep* 2002;3:301-6
- Management of STI syndromes in men. In: Holmes KK, Mårdh PA, Sparling PF, Lemon S, Stamm W, Piot P, et al. *Sexually transmitted diseases*. 3rd ed. New York: McGraw Hill, 1999:833-71
- Morton RS, ed. *Gonorrhoea* 3rd ed. London: WB Saunders, 1977
- Ostrow DG, Sandholzer TA, and Felman YM, eds. *Homosexual men: diagnosis, treatment, and research*. New York: Plenum, 1983

6 Other conditions of the male genital tract commonly seen in sexually transmitted infection clinics

John Richens

Conditions affecting the glans and prepuce

The glans and prepuce are susceptible to many local and generalised skin conditions. Mild irritation often responds to simple advice to avoid soap, wash with a weak salt solution, and use emollients. A number of other conditions respond to topical steroid treatment. Persistent conditions may require biopsy because a number of chronic skin conditions of the glans can undergo malignant transformation. The insertion of rings through the urethral meatus (the "Prince Albert") has become popular in recent years. Such rings rarely give rise to local infections; however, infections are more likely to be associated with anal rings.

Infectious conditions

Candida balanoposthitis can produce soreness, pruritus, erythema, and fissuring. Dry, dull, red, glazed plaques and papules, sometimes eroded, may be seen. The condition is often linked to diabetes. Treatment with an imidazole cream (see Chapter 20) is recommended, together with advice to avoid soap and to bathe with water. Treatment of infected partners has not been shown to benefit men or women with symptomatic *Candida* infection.

Bacterial infections

Purulent infections of the glans are most often seen in uncircumcised males with phimosis. Important organisms involved include anaerobes, streptococci, staphylococci, and *Gardnerella*. Treatment according to microbiological reports is recommended. When a foul smelling discharge is present, anaerobic infection is likely and treatment with metronidazole 400 mg twice daily for one week is recommended.

Dermatoses of the glans penis

Any persistent lesion that fails to respond to simple measures should undergo biopsy. Three histologically similar forms of penile intraepithelial neoplasia (carcinoma in situ) of the male genitalia have been described. They are the erythroplasia of Queyrat, which produces velvety plaques on the glans, Bowen's disease, characterised by erythematous plaques on the shaft or more proximally, and Bowenoid papulosis, which produces multiple lesions after infection with human papilloma virus type 16. Lichen sclerosus (in men sometimes called balanitis xerotica obliterans) produces striking white patches on the glans that may undergo malignant transformation. Treatment is with strong topical steroids and, occasionally, circumcision and meatotomy for cases complicated by phimosis and meatal stricture. Other steroid responsive conditions of the glans are plasma cell (Zoon's) balanitis, which produces

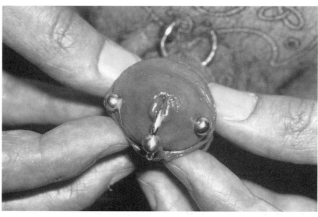
Ring through the urethal meatus

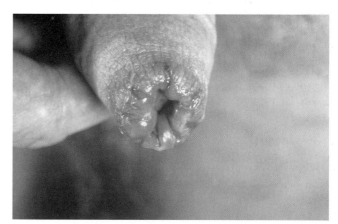
Candida balanitis

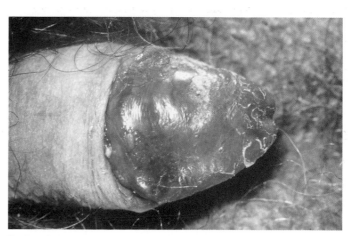
Erythroplasia of Queyrat

painless red-orange coloured plaques with "cayenne pepper" spots, lichen planus, psoriasis, and seborrhoeic dermatitis, clues to which are found in the presence of characteristic lesions at other body sites, and circinate balanitis, which is characterised by "geographical" areas of erythema on the glans with white margins. It is linked to other features of Reiter's syndrome. Fixed drug eruptions occasionally are confined to the penis, the best known cause being the tetracyclines.

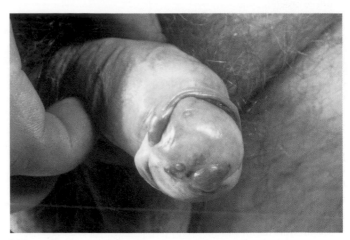

Lichen sclerosus

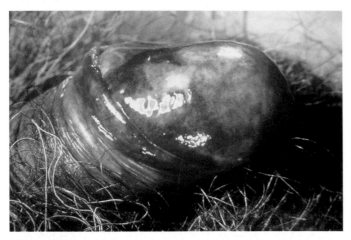

Zoon's balanitis

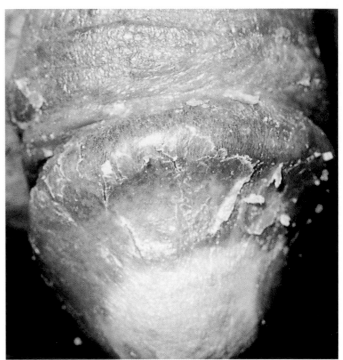

Psoriasis

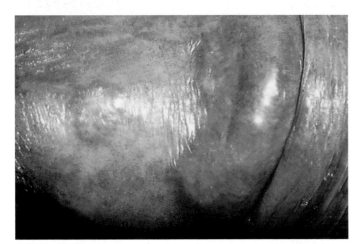

Lichen planus

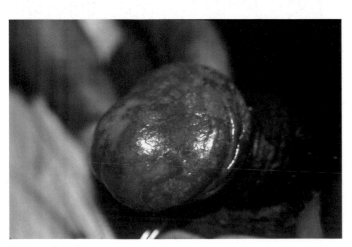

Circinate balanitis

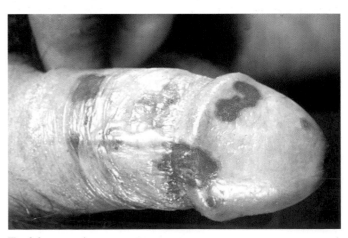

Fixed drug eruptions

Phimosis, paraphimosis, and lymphocoele

A painful inability to retract the prepuce can result from any chronic inflammatory condition of the prepuce. The condition can be relieved by application of topical steroids or surgical means. Paraphimosis results from prolonged retraction of the prepuce, which leads to constriction of the distal shaft and oedema of the glans. In the early stages, the prepuce can be pushed back by applying firm pressure. This is made easier by first reducing the swelling with ice packs, compression bandaging, or local injections of hyaluronidase. Late cases may require multiple needle puncture and expression of fluid under local anaesthetic (Dundee technique) or surgical intervention.

The term lymphocoele is used to describe a lesion of unknown aetiology that feels like a transverse thrombosed lymphatic vessel close to the corona. This harmless condition develops quite quickly (often after vigorous sex) and resolves spontaneously, usually in a few days.

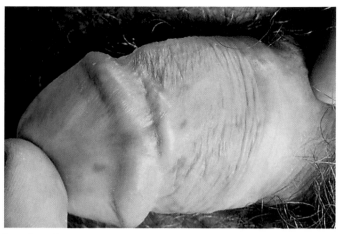
Lymphocoele

Common lesions of scrotal skin

Angiokeratomas are harmless small papules with a deep-red or purplish colour, which increase in number with age. Multiple epidermal (sebaceous) cysts are sometimes observed on the scrotum. These conditions are usually left untreated.

Tinea cruris and erythrasma

Tinea cruris is a superficial fungal infection that affects the skin of the groin; it is seen mostly in men. Patients complain of soreness and itching. Examination shows a well demarcated discoloration of the affected skin. Fungal hyphae can be seen in skin scrapings. Treatment with topical or oral imidazole drugs clears the infection.

Erythrasma is a bacterial condition caused by *Corynebacterium minutissimum*. It occurs in the same area as tinea cruris but tends to have a browner colour and a less well demarcated edge. Porphyrins produced by the bacteria give the lesion a coral pink colour when viewed by Wood's light. It can be treated with erythromycin.

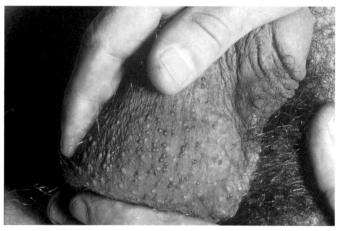
Angiokeratoma

Semen abnormalities

The observation of blood in the ejaculate causes considerable anxiety. The great majority of cases settle quickly and no underlying disease is detected. A screen for sexually transmitted infections (STIs), urinalysis, examination of prostate, and a blood pressure check are advised. Further investigation is only indicated if symptoms persist. It very occasionally can be associated with hypertension or rare conditions involving the male genital tract in older men. Abnormal lumpiness of semen has been described in patients infected with *Schistosoma haematobium*. A history of exposure to potentially contaminated water in tropical areas should be followed by investigation for schistosomiasis. Patients with prostatis sometimes complain of changes in semen colour or consistency or ejaculatory pain. It is common to encounter individuals from South Asia who are convinced that they are losing semen unnaturally, giving rise to feelings of lethargy and tiredness. This condition is known as "dhat" in India and is sometimes dignified with the pseudoscientific name "prostatorrhoea." It is closely bound up with cultural concepts of semen and vitality and has no identifiable organic basis.

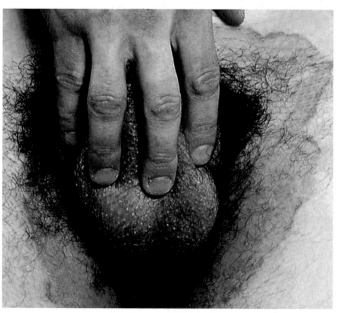
Tinea cruris

Peyronie's disease

Fibrosis in the tunica albuginea of the penile shaft can give rise to deformity, which is accentuated during erection. Patients complain of deformity and sometimes pain and difficulty with intercourse. The diagnosis is made by palpating thick fibrous plaques in the penile shaft. Surgery may be required for some patients.

Disorders of male sexual function

A study of new heterosexual male attenders at a London genitourinary medicine clinic in London in 1997 found that 24% of patients reported sexual dysfunction. Disorders of sexual function are often psychological; however, neurological, endocrinological, and other disorders contribute to a considerable proportion of cases of erectile dysfunction.

Sexually transmitted infections rarely interfere directly with sexual function, although concerns about STIs or HIV often are expressed by patients with dysfunction. Loss of libido and erectile dysfunction are reported commonly by men infected with HIV and may be exacerbated by antiviral treatment.

Once an individual has experienced sexual dysfunction, performance anxiety readily develops, which exacerbates the problem. Reducing performance anxiety is a key aim of psychological therapies.

Erectile dysfunction

Patients complain of failure to achieve or maintain an erection. Psychological factors can be identified by careful history taking. If the patient does not experience spontaneous erections on waking and cannot masturbate to orgasm, an organic disease is more likely.

Patients should be evaluated carefully for the possibility of organic disease, including measurement of blood pressure, genital examination, and, in some cases, peripheral pulse and neurological examinations. Screening for diabetes and dipstick urinalysis is recommended for all patients. In selected cases, measuring free plasma testosterone (patients with small testes or who report low libido), blood lipids, haemoglobin electrophoresis, follicle stimulating hormone, luteinising hormone, prolactin, thyroid, renal, and liver function tests, or vascular imaging may be indicated.

Treatment options (for which guidelines have recently been published in the *BMJ*) include psychosexual counselling, intracavernosal or intraurethral alprostadil, or oral sildenafil. Mechanical devices and surgical treatments are used occasionally. Treatment should be supervised by specialist centres that can arrange prompt referral for dangerous (albeit rare) complications of therapy, such as priapism.

Premature ejaculation

An organic cause is unlikely to be found. Therapy is usually behavioural and involves training the patient to delay ejaculation by using a variety of graduated stop-start exercises first, alone, using masturbatory exercises, and then with a partner.

The best known approach with partners is the "sensate focus" technique pioneered by Masters and Johnson, which initially prohibits genital contact and progresses gradually to more intimate contact as more control is achieved. As an alternative, clomipramine and other antidepressants can be taken four to six hours before intercourse with some benefit.

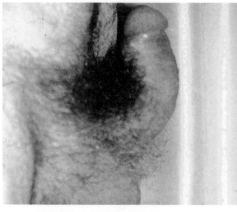

Peyronie's disease caused by the presence of a dorsal plaque in the penis. Reproduced from Tomlinson J(ed) *ABC of sexual health*

Conditions that can cause disorders of male sexual function

- Hypertension
- Sickle cell disease
- Vascular disease (for example, Leriche syndrome)
- Diabetes
- Neurological disease (for example, multiple sclerosis)
- Endocrine disease (for example, deficiencies of testosterone, gonadotrophins, hypothyroidism, and prolactinoma)
- Alcoholism and substance abuse
- Liver and kidney diseases
- Adverse effects of drugs (for example, antihypertensive and antidepressant medication)
- After prostate and abdominal surgery

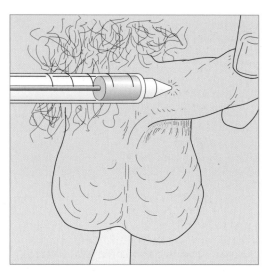

Intracavernosal injection of alprostadil. Reproduced from Tomlinson J (ed) *ABC of sexual health*

Further reading

- Chadda RK. Dhat syndrome: is it a distinct clinical entity? A study of illness behaviour characteristics. *Acta Psychiatr Scand* 1995;9:136-9
- Edwards S. Balanitis and balanoposthitis: a review. *Genitourin Med* 1996;72:155-9
- McKenna G, Schousboe M, Paltridge G. Subjective change in ejaculate as symptom of infection with *Schistosoma haematobium* in travellers. *BMJ* 1997;315:1000-1
- McMillan A. Lymphocoele and localized lymphoedema of the penis. *Br J Vener Dis* 1976;52:409
- Reynard JM, Barua JM. Reduction of paraphimosis the simple way: the Dundee technique. *Br J Urol* 1999;83:859-86
- Tomlinson J. *ABC of sexual health*. London: BMJ Publishing Group, 1999

7 Vaginal discharge—causes, diagnosis, and treatment

Helen Mitchell

Vaginal discharge is a common presenting symptom seen by doctors in many services (primary care, gynaecology, family planning, and departments of genitourinary medicine (GUM)). Vaginal discharge may be physiological or pathological. Although abnormal vaginal discharge often prompts women to seek screening for sexually transmitted infections (STIs), vaginal discharge is poorly predictive of the presence of an STI. This chapter focuses on the causes and diagnosis of vaginal discharge and treatment of the most common infective causes.

Aetiology

Physiological discharge

Normal vaginal flora (lactobacilli) colonise the vaginal epithelium and may play a role in defence against infection. They maintain the normal vaginal pH between 3.8 and 4.4. The quality and quantity of vaginal discharge may alter in the same woman in cycles and over time; each woman has her own sense of normality and what is acceptable or excessive for her.

Pathological vaginal discharge

Vulvovaginal candidiasis is a common infective cause of vaginal discharge that affects about 75% of women at some time during their reproductive life, with 40-50% having two or more episodes. Bacterial vaginosis is one of the most common diagnoses in women attending GUM clinics. As 50% of cases of bacterial vaginosis are asymptomatic, the true prevalence of this condition in the community is uncertain. Bacterial vaginosis is associated with a new sexual partner and frequent change of sexual partners. A reduced rate of bacterial vaginosis is seen among women in monogamous sexual relationships, but it can occur in virginal women. Increased rates of bacterial vaginosis occur in certain groups of women, such as black African women, lesbians, and smokers.

Recurrence of bacterial vaginosis after treatment is common and can be increased by personal hygiene practices, such as vaginal douching, that disrupt the normal vaginal flora. Bacterial vaginosis may also be associated with concurrent STIs, commonly *Trichomonas vaginalis*. Bacterial vaginosis is associated with pelvic infection after induced abortion and in pregnancy with pre-term delivery and low birth weight (see Chapter 9). Trichomoniasis is less common in affluent countries but reaches high levels (often 10-20%) among poor women in developing countries as well as among disadvantaged women in affluent countries. Although vulvovaginal candidiasis and bacterial vaginosis often develop independently of sexual activity, trichomoniasis is mainly sexually transmitted and has been ranked by the World Health Organization as the most prevalent non-viral STI in the world, with an estimated 172 million new cases per annum.

What may influence physiological discharge?

Age
- Pre-pubertal
- Reproductive
- Post-menopausal

Hormones
- Hormonal contraception
- Cyclical hormonal changes
- Pregnancy

Local factors
- Menstruation
- Post partum
- Malignancy
- Semen
- Personal habits and hygiene

Pathological vaginal discharge

Infective discharge

Common causes
- Organisms
  - *Candida albicans*
  - Bacterial vaginosis
  - *Trichomonas vaginalis*
  - *Chlamydia trachomatis*
  - *Neisseria gonorrhoeae*
- Infective conditions
  - Acute pelvic inflammatory disease (see Chapter 8)
  - Post-operative pelvic infection
  - Post-abortal sepsis
  - Puerperal sepsis

Less common causes
- Human papillomavirus
- Primary syphilis
- *Mycoplasma genitalium*
- *Ureaplasma urealyticum*
- *Escherichia coli*

Other conditions

Common causes
- Retained tampon or condom
- Chemical irritation
- Allergic responses
- Ectropion
- Endocervical polyp
- Intrauterine device in situ
- Atrophic changes

Less common causes
- Physical trauma
- Vault granulation tissue
- Vesicovaginal fistula
- Rectovaginal fistula
- Neoplasia

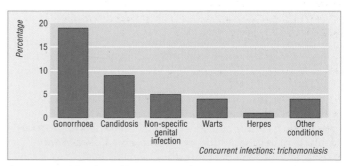

Concurrent STIs found in a survey of women with *T vaginalis*

Overview of genital candidiasis and bacterial vaginosis

Genital candidiasis

Cause
- *Candida albicans* in 80-95% of cases; *C glabrata* in about 5%

Associated conditions
- Diabetes mellitus, pregnancy, antibiotic usage, and immunosuppression

Transmission
- Mostly non-sexual

Site of infection
- Vulva, vagina, glans, prepuce, and rectum

Symptoms in women
- Vulvar pruritus, white curdy discharge with "cottage cheese" appearance and sour milk odour, external dysuria, and superficial dyspareunia

Symptoms in men
- Soreness, pruritus, redness, and fissuring of glans and prepuce

Examination findings in women
- Redness, fissuring, excoriation of vulva, swelling of labia, intertrigo, and lichenification. Thick, white, adherent discharge with vaginal wall erythema

Examination findings in men
- Dry, dull, red, glazed plaques and papules on glans and prepuce

Main methods of detection
- Fungal hyphae and budding yeasts in smears and culture

Recommended intravaginal treatments for women
- Treatment regimes offer 80-95% clinical and mycological cure rates in acute vulvovaginal candidiasis in non-pregnant women
- Vaginal
  - Butoconazole 2% cream 5 g for one to three days (C)
  - Clotrimazole pessary 500 mg single dose (C, E, U, W), 200 mg for three days (C, E, W), or 100 mg for six to seven days (C, U, W)
  - Econazole pessary 150 mg for one to three days (U)
  - Miconazole ovule 1.2 g single dose (E, U)
- Recurrent infection
  - Nystatin vaginal pessary 1-200 000 units for two weeks (C, U) or fluconazole 100 mg per week (see recurrent vaginal *Candida*)
- Recommended oral therapies
  - Fluconazole 150 mg single dose (C, E, U, W)
  - Itraconazole 200 mg twice daily for one day (E, U)
- Topical symptomatic relief suitable for both sexes
  - Clotrimazole 1% cream
  - Miconazole nitrate 2%
  - Clotrimazole 1% with 1% hydrocortisone
- A large number of other preparations are available

Bacterial vaginosis

Cause
- Bacterial vaginosis has a polymicrobial aetiology. Organisms involved in the aetiology of bacterial vaginosis include anaerobes *Mobiluncus* sp. and *Prevotella* sp., *Gardnerella vaginalis*, and *Mycoplasma hominis*

Main symptoms
- Vaginal discharge with fishy odour that increases after unprotected sexual intercourse and with menstruation

Main methods of diagnosis
- Amsel's diagnostic criteria (three out of four of these criteria need to be present to diagnose bacterial vaginosis)
  - Vaginal pH >4.5
  - Homogeneous grey vaginal discharge
  - 10% potassium hydroxide produces fishy odour "whiff test"
  - Clue cells present on wet mount
- Nugent's diagnostic criteria (see Chapter 17)
- Note that culture for *Gardnerella* is no longer a recommended approach to diagnosis

Recommended treatments
- Treatment regimes have similar cure rates of 70-80% after four weeks. Compliance with therapy may result in a symptomatic cure but not a microbiological cure, so relapse after single dose metronidazole (2 g) treatment is common; 60% of women relapse in three months
- Clindamycin is effective but also kills lactobacilli, and topical treatment may predispose patient to vulvovaginal candidiasis. Intravaginal clindamycin can cause condom failure
- Metronidazole 2 g single dose (C (2), E (2), U, W (2))
- Metronidazole 400 mg twice daily for five to seven days (C, E, U, W)
- Metronidazole 0.75% gel daily for five days (C, E, U, W (2))
- Clindamycin 2% cream 5 g daily for seven days (C, E, U, W (2))
- Clindamycin ovules 100 mg daily for three days (C)
- Clindamycin 300 mg orally twice daily for seven days (C, E, W (2))
- Prophylaxis for surgical interventions: rectal metronidazole 1 g or intravenous metronidazole 500 mg

C = Centers for Disease Control, USA; E = European STI guidelines; U = UK National Guidelines; W = World Health Organization, (2) = second line recommendation.

Principles of management

As mentioned, self reported symptoms and the clinical appearance of vaginal discharge are both very variable and do not permit accurate determination of the presence or absence of a specific STI. If a full screen to exclude STIs is not carried out this, may lead to delayed diagnosis and possible long term complications.

An assessment of an individual woman's STI risk can be made by taking a sexual history. A practitioner working in a primary care setting can then decide whether it is appropriate to refer a woman with identified risk factors in her history directly to a GUM clinic for further management.

The advantage of managing vaginal discharge in a GUM clinic is that full microbiological tests are done to establish an accurate diagnosis. Microscopy is also carried out routinely for symptomatic cases, so an immediate diagnosis will be available for many women.

Questions to ask women who complain of vaginal discharge

Discharge	Associated symptoms
• Onset	• Itching
• Duration	• Soreness
• Amount	• Dysuria
• Colour	• Intermenstrual or post-coital bleeding
• Blood staining	• Lower abdominal pain
• Consistency	• Pelvic pain
• Odour	• Dyspareunia—superficial and deep
• Previous episodes	

Risk factors for presence of STIs

- Age under 25 years
- No condom use
- Symptoms developed after recent change of sexual partner or multiple contacts
- Recurrent or persistent symptoms
- Symptoms in partner
- Symptoms imply complications
- Partner's risk behaviour